Slow Cooker Cookbook for Your Breakfast

Tasty and Affordable Slow Cooker Recipes to Start Your Day with the Right Foot

Sean Miller

© Copyright 2020 - All rights reserved.

The content contained within this book may not be reproduced, duplicated or transmitted without direct written permission from the author or the publisher.

Under no circumstances will any blame or legal responsibility be held against the publisher, or author, for any damages, reparation, or monetary loss due to the information contained within this book. Either directly or indirectly.

Legal Notice:

This book is copyright protected. This book is only for personal use. You cannot amend, distribute, sell, use, quote or paraphrase any part, or the content within this book, without the consent of the author or publisher.

Disclaimer Notice:

Please note the information contained within this document is for educational and entertainment purposes only. All effort has been executed to present accurate, up to date, and reliable, complete information. No warranties of any kind are declared or implied. Readers acknowledge that the author is not engaging in the rendering of legal, financial, medical or professional advice. The content within this book has been derived from various sources. Please consult a licensed professional before attempting any techniques outlined in this book.

By reading this document, the reader agrees that under no circumstances is the author responsible for any losses, direct or indirect, which are incurred as a result of the use of information contained within this document, including, but not limited to, ― errors, omissions, or inaccuracies.

Table of Contents

Zucchini & Spinach with Bacon ... 6

Pepperoni Pizza with Meat Crust ... 8

Spinach & Sausage Pizza ... 10

Greek-Style Frittata with Spinach and Feta Cheese ... 13

Nut & Zucchini Bread ... 15

Cheese & Cauliflower Bake ... 17

Ham & Cheese Broccoli Brunch Bowl ... 20

Eggplant & Sausage Bake ... 22

Three-Cheese Artichoke Hearts Bake ... 24

Sweet Ham Maple Breakfast ... 26

Sausage Casserole Breakfast ... 28

Mushroom Bacon Breakfast ... 30

Zucchini Cinnamon Nut Bread ... 33

Ham and Spinach Frittata ... 35

Cheese Grits ... 37

Pineapple Cake with Pecans ... 39

Potato Casserole for Breakfast ... 41

Cinnamon Rolls ... 43

Quinoa Pie ... 45

Quinoa Muffins with Peanut Butter ... 47

Veggie Omelets ... 49

Apple Pie with Oatmeal ... 51

Vanilla French Toast ... 53

Greek Eggs Casserole ... 55

Banana Bread ... 57

Treacle Sponge with Honey	59
Sticky Pecan Buns with Maple	61
Vegetarian Pot Pie	63
Blueberry Porridge	65
Cauliflower and Eggs Bowls	67
Milk Oatmeal	69
Asparagus Egg Casserole	71
Vanilla Maple Oats	73
Raspberry Oatmeal	75
Pork and Eggplant Casserole	77
Baby Spinach Rice Mix	79
Baby Carrots in Syrup	81
Green Muffins	83
Scallions and Bacon Omelet	85
Cowboy Breakfast Casserole	87
Maple Banana Oatmeal	89
Potato Muffins	91
Eggs and Sweet Potato Mix	93
Veggie Hash Brown Mix	95
Coconut Cranberry Quinoa	97
Scrambled Eggs in Ramekins	99
Enchilada Breakfast Casserole	101
White Chocolate Oatmeal	103
Bacon-Wrapped Hotdogs	105
Apple Granola Crumble	107

Zucchini & Spinach with Bacon

Preparation time:

10 minutes

Cooking time:

6 hours

Servings: 4 people

Ingredients:

- 8 slices bacon
- 1 tablespoon olive oil
- 4 medium zucchinis, cubed
- 2 cups baby spinach
- 1 red onion, diced
- 6 garlic cloves, sliced thin
- 1 cup chicken broth
- salt and pepper to taste

Directions:

1. Warm-up olive oil in a pan, brown the bacon for 5 minutes.
2. Break it into pieces in the pan.
3. Place remaining ingredients in the slow cooker, pour the bacon and fat from the pan

over the fixing inside the slow cooker. Cover, cook on low for 6 hours.

Nutrition:
- Calories: 290
- Carbs: 16g
- Fat: 20g
- Protein: 12g

Pepperoni Pizza with Meat Crust

Preparation time:

5 minutes

Cooking time:

4 hours

Servings: 4 people

Ingredients:

- 2.2. pounds lean ground beef
- 2 garlic cloves, minced
- 1 tablespoon dry, fried onions
- salt and pepper to taste
- 2 cups shredded mozzarella
- 1 ¾ cup sugarless ready-made pizza sauce
- 2 cups shredded yellow cheese, cheddar
- ½ cup sliced pepperoni

Directions:

1. Brown the beef with the seasoning in a pan.
2. Mix the beef with the cheese.
3. Butter the slow cooker and spread the crust out evenly over the bottom.

4. Pour the pizza sauce over the crust and spread evenly. Top with the cheese and arrange the pepperoni slices.
5. Cover, cook on low for 4 hours. Serve.

Nutrition:
- Calories: 320
- Carbs: 31g
- Fat: 16g
- Protein: 15g

Spinach & Sausage Pizza

Preparation time:

5 minutes

Cooking time:

6 hours

Servings:

4 people

Ingredients:

- 1 tablespoon olive oil
- 1 cup lean ground beef
- 2 cups spicy pork sausage
- 2 garlic cloves, minced
- 1 tablespoon dry, fried onions
- salt and pepper to taste
- 1 ¾ cups sugarless ready-made pizza sauce
- 3 cups fresh spinach
- ½ cup sliced pepperoni
- ¼ cup pitted black olives, sliced
- ¼ cup sun-dried tomatoes, chopped
- ½ cup spring onions, chopped
- 3 cups shredded mozzarella

Directions:

1. In a pan, heat the olive oil. Brown the beef, then the pork.
2. Drain the oil off the meat, then mix.
3. Pour the meat into the slow cooker.
4. Spread evenly and press down.
5. Alternate in layers the pizza sauce, toppings, and cheese.
6. Cover and cook on low within 4-6 hours. Serve.

Nutrition:

- Calories: 314
- Carbs: 34 g
- Fat: 12 g
- Protein: 17 g

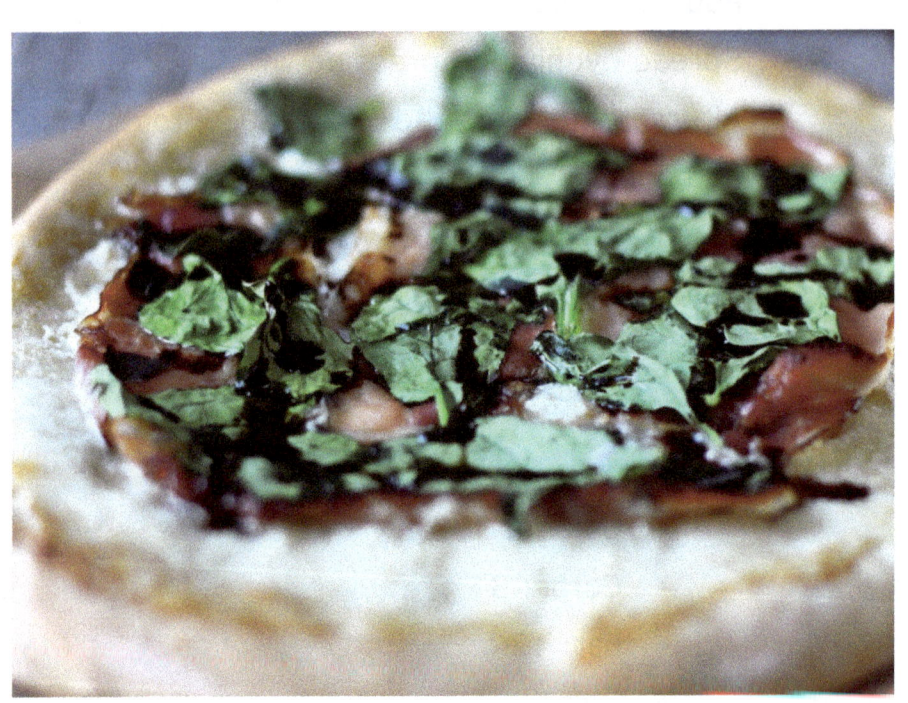

Greek-Style Frittata with Spinach and Feta Cheese

Preparation time:
10 minutes
Cooking time:
4 hours
Servings:
4 people

Ingredients:
- 2 cups spinach, fresh or frozen
- 8 eggs, lightly beaten
- 1 cup plain yogurt
- 1 small onion, cut into small pieces
- 2 red roasted peppers, peeled
- 1 garlic clove, crushed
- 1 cup feta cheese, crumbled
- 2 tablespoons softened butter
- 2 tablespoons olive oil
- salt and pepper to taste
- 1 teaspoon dried oregano

Directions:

1. Sauté the onion and garlic for 5 minutes.
2. Add the spinach, heat for an additional 2 minutes. Let the mixture cool down.
3. Roast the red peppers in a dry pan or under the broiler.
4. Peel them and cut them into small pieces.
5. Beat the eggs, yogurt, and seasoning in a separate bowl.
6. Combine well.
7. Add the peppers and the onion mixture. Mix again.
8. Crumble the feta cheese using a fork, add it to the frittata.
9. Grease the bottom and sides of the slow cooker with butter. Pour the mixture into it. Cover, cook on low for 4 hours.

Nutrition:

- Calories: 206
- Carbs: 13 g
- Fat: 13 g
- Protein: 11 g

Nut & Zucchini Bread

Preparation time:

10 minutes

Cooking time:

3 hours

Servings:

4 people

Ingredients:

- 2 cups shredded zucchini
- ½ cup ground walnuts
- 1 cup ground almonds
- 1/3 cup coconut flakes
- 2 teaspoons cinnamon
- ½ teaspoon baking soda
- 1 ½ teaspoons baking powder
- ½ teaspoon salt
- 3 large eggs
- 1/3 cup softened coconut oil
- 1 cup sweetener, Swerve (or a suitable substitute)
- 2 teaspoons vanilla

Directions:
1. Shred the zucchini and ground the walnuts. In a bowl, beat the eggs, oil, sweetener, and vanilla together.
2. Add the dry ingredients to the wet mixture. Fold in the zucchini and walnuts.
3. Pour the batter into your bread pan, which fits inside the slow cooker.
4. Crumble aluminum foil into four balls, place on the bottom of the slow cooker, and set the pan in the slow cooker with a paper towel on top to absorb the water—cook on high for 3 hours.
5. Cool, wrap in foil, and refrigerate.
6. Serve cold with tea or coffee.

Nutrition:
- Calories: 90
- Carbs: 12g
- Fat: 4g
- Protein: 1g

Cheese & Cauliflower Bake

Preparation time:

5 minutes

Cooking time:

4 hours

Servings:

4 people

Ingredients:

- 1 head cauliflower, cut into florets
- ½ cup cream cheese
- ¼ cup whipping cream
- 2 tablespoons lard or butter
- 1 tablespoon lard or butter to grease the slow cooker
- 1 teaspoon salt
- ½ teaspoon fresh ground black pepper
- ½ cup yellow cheese, cheddar, shredded
- 6 slices of bacon, crisped and crumbled

Directions:

1. Grease the slow cooker.

2. Add all the fixing, except the cheese and the bacon.
3. Cook on low for 3 hours.
4. Open the lid and add cheese.
5. Re-cover, cook for an additional hour.
6. Top with the bacon and serve.

Tip:

Good for brunch with a couple of cherry tomatoes and avocado slices.

Nutrition:

- Calories: 178
- Carbs: 8g
- Fat: 11g
- Protein: 5g

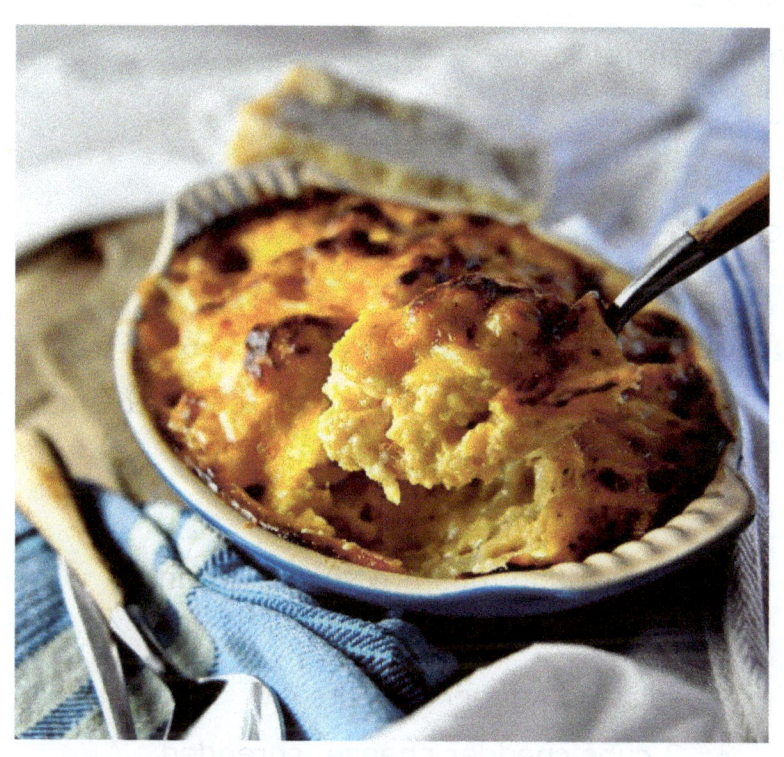

Ham & Cheese Broccoli Brunch Bowl

Preparation time:

5 minutes

Cooking time:

8 hours

Servings:

4 people

Ingredients:

- 1 medium head of broccoli, chopped small
- 4 cups vegetable broth
- 2 tablespoons olive oil
- 1 teaspoon mustard seeds, ground
- 3 garlic cloves, minced
- salt and pepper to taste
- 2 cups cheddar cheese, shredded
- 2 cups ham, cubed
- pinch of paprika

Directions:

1. Add all ingredients to the 6-quart slow cooker in order of the list. Cover, cook on low for 8 hours.

Nutrition:

- Calories: 320
- Carbs: 28g
- Fat: 17g
- Protein: 14g

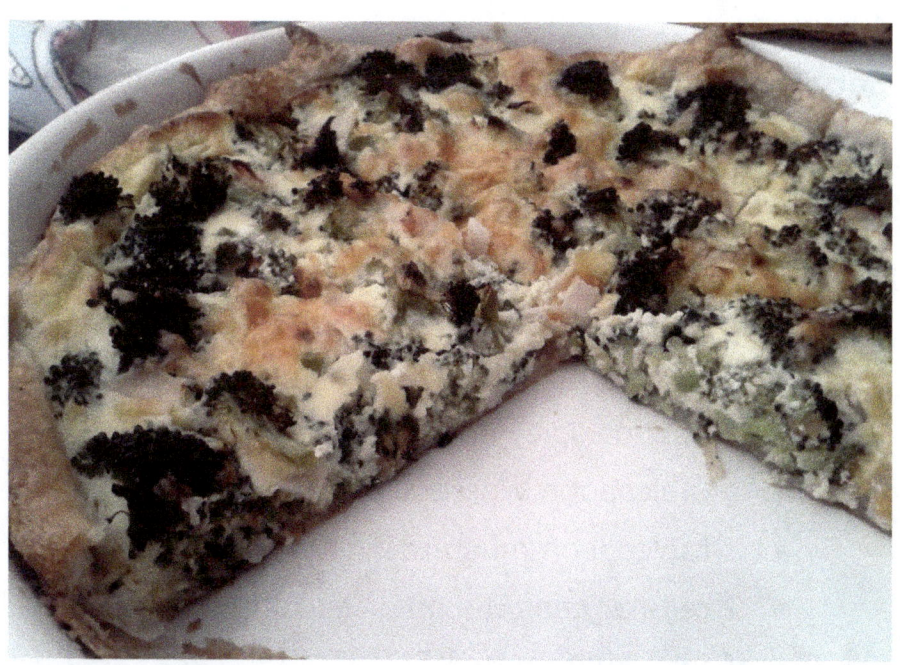

Eggplant & Sausage Bake

Preparation time:

10 minutes

Cooking time:

4 hours

Servings:

4 people

Ingredients:

- 2 cups eggplant, cubed, salted, and drained
- 1 tablespoon olive oil
- 2 pounds spicy pork sausage
- 1 tablespoon Worcestershire sauce
- 1 tablespoon mustard
- 2 regular cans Italian diced tomatoes
- 1 jar tomato passata
- 2 cups mozzarella cheese, shredded

Directions:

1. Grease the slow cooker with olive oil. Mix the sausage, Worcestershire sauce, and mustard. Pour the mixture into the slow cooker.
2. Top the meat mixture with eggplant.

3. Pour the tomatoes over the batter, sprinkle with grated cheese.
4. Cover, cook on low for 4 hours. Enjoy for brunch.

Nutrition:
- Calories: 345
- Carbs: 34g
- Fat: 15g
- Protein: 21g

Three-Cheese Artichoke Hearts Bake

Preparation time:

5 minutes

Cooking time:

2 hours

Servings:

4 people

Ingredients:

- 1 cup cheddar cheese, grated
- ½ cup dry parmesan cheese
- 1 cup cream cheese
- 1 cup spinach, chopped
- 1 clove of garlic, crushed
- 1 jar artichoke hearts, chopped
- salt and pepper to taste

Directions:

1. Place all the ingredients in the 6-quart slow cooker. Mix lightly.
2. Cover, cook on high for 2 hours. Serve.

Nutrition:

- Calories: 40
- Carbs: 7 g
- Fat: 0 g
- Protein: 2 g

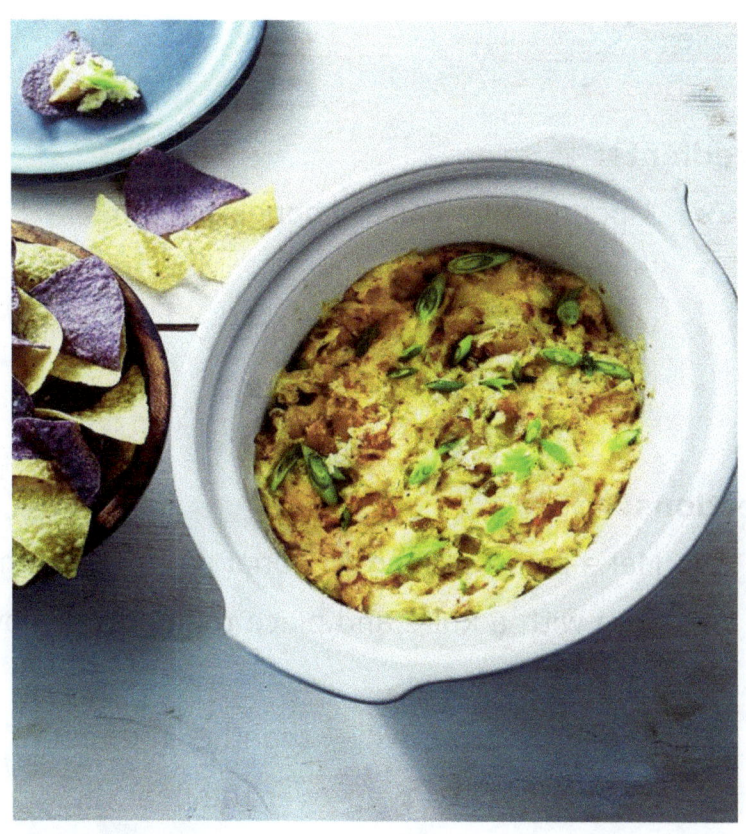

Sweet Ham Maple Breakfast

Preparation time:

15 minutes

Cooking time:

3-4 hours

Servings:

4 people

Ingredients:

- 3-pound fully-cooked boneless ham
- ½ cup of maple syrup
- ½ cup of Honey Dijon Mustard
- ½ cup of packed brown sugar

Directions:

1. Make cross-shaped diagonal patterns on the ham with a knife and place them into a slow cooker.
2. In a large bowl, whisk together the rest of the ingredients and pour over the ham.
3. Cover and cook on low within 3-4 hours. Take the ham out and cover with foil for 10 minutes. Slice and serve.

Nutrition:

- Calories: 430
- Fat: 24 g
- Protein: 32 g
- Carbs: 13 g

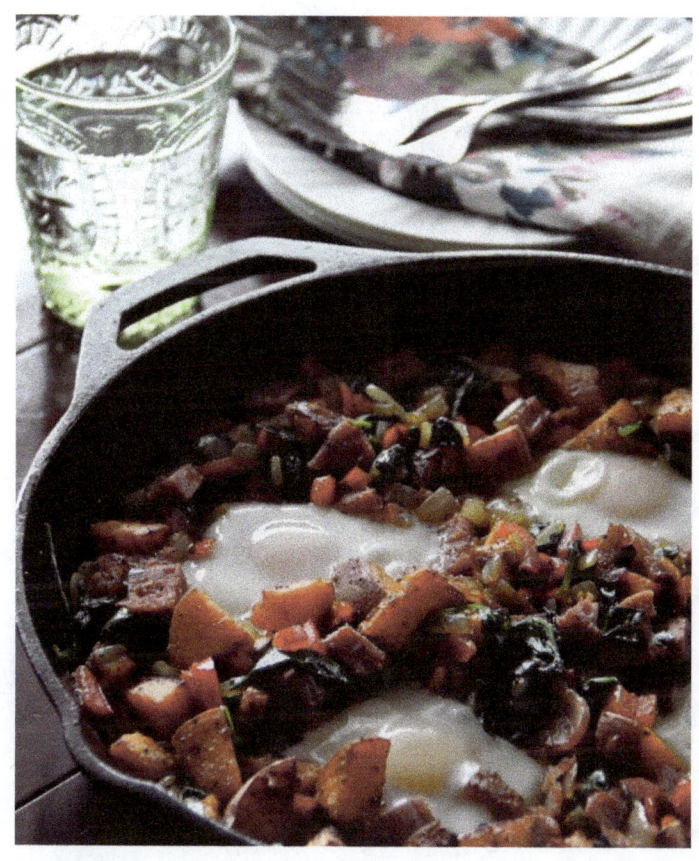

Sausage Casserole Breakfast

Preparation time:

15 minutes

Cooking time:

4-5 hours

Servings:

4 people

Ingredients:

- 8 large eggs
- 1 ½ cups of low-fat milk
- 1 pound of cooked bulk sausage, drained
- 1 seeded and chopped jalapeño
- 1 chopped red bell pepper
- ¾ cup sliced green onions
- 2 cups of low-fat Mexican blend cheese
- 9 corn tortillas
- ½ cup of salsa

Directions:

1. Mix the eggs, jalapeño, and milk in a large bowl. In another large bowl, combine the

cheese, green onions, sausage, and red bell pepper.
2. Arrange 3 tortillas on the base of a greased slow cooker.
3. Spread a layer of the sausage mixture over the tortillas.
4. Repeat the layering, and then pour the egg mixture over the top.
5. Cover and cook on low within 4-5 hours.
6. Divide onto plates and serve with the salsa.

Nutrition:
- Calories: 386
- Fat: 24g
- Fiber: 2.6g
- Protein: 24.7g

Mushroom Bacon Breakfast

Preparation time:

15 minutes

Cooking time:

4-6 hours

Servings:

4 people

Ingredients:

- 2 cups of ground sausage, cooked
- ½ cup of chopped onion
- 1 tablespoon of dried parsley
- 1 teaspoon of garlic powder
- 1 teaspoon of thyme
- 6 slices of bacon, cooked and crumbled
- 2 cups of organic chicken broth
- 1 red bell pepper, chopped
- ½ cup of parmesan cheese
- 1 cup of heavy cream
- 2 cups of sliced mushrooms
- Salt and black pepper

Directions:
1. Place all of the fixings into a large slow cooker. Cook within 4-6 hours on a low setting.
2. Ensure that you don't overcook the ingredients or cook the food at too high heat.
3. It will cause the cream to separate.
4. When the food is cooked, divide onto plates and serve hot.

Nutrition:
- Calories: 166
- Carbs: 2.1g
- Fat: 15.5g
- Fiber: 0.3 g
- Protein: 6.7 g

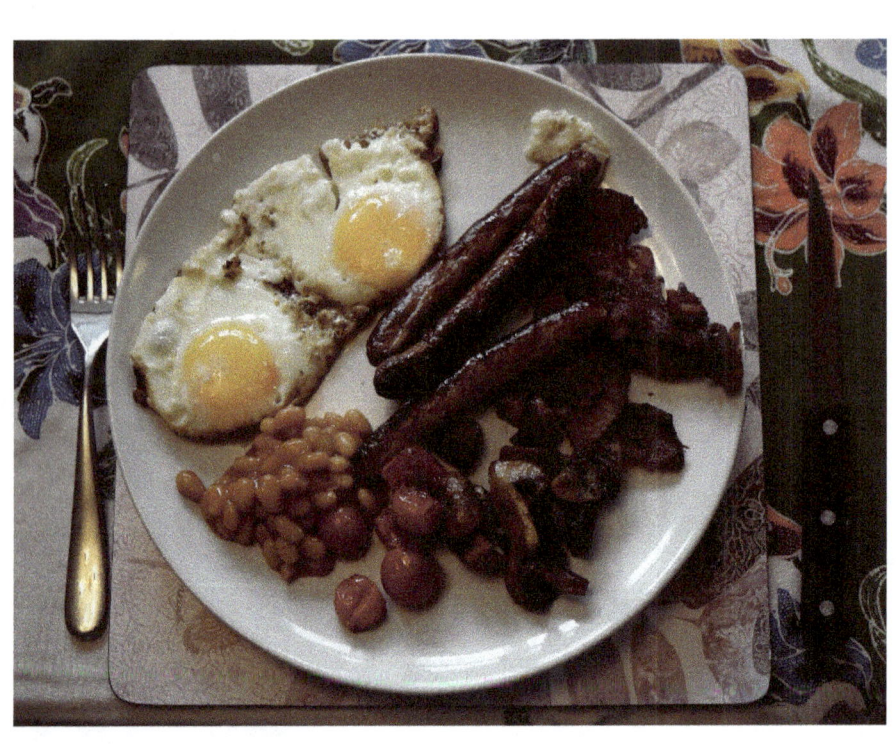

Zucchini Cinnamon Nut Bread

Preparation time:

15 minutes

Cooking time:

3 hours

Servings:

4 people

Ingredients:

- 2 cups of zucchini, shredded
- ½ cup of ground walnuts
- 1 cup of ground almonds
- 1/3 cup of coconut flakes
- 2 teaspoons of cinnamon
- ½ teaspoon of baking soda
- 1 ½ teaspoon of baking powder
- ½ teaspoon of salt
- 3 large eggs
- 1/3 cup of softened coconut oil
- 1 cup of sweetener of your choice
- 2 teaspoons of vanilla

Directions:
1. In a large bowl, beat the vanilla, sweetener, oil, and eggs and whisk them together thoroughly.
2. Add all of the dry fixings to the egg mixture. Add the walnuts and the zucchini.
3. You will need a bread pan that is small enough to fit into the slow cooker.
4. Pour the batter into it.
5. Roll up aluminum foil into four balls and set them on the base of the slow cooker.
6. Put the pan into your slow cooker and place a paper towel over the top to absorb condensation.
7. Cook on high for 3 hours.
8. Allow the bread to cool down, wrap it in foil and place it in the fridge. Serve cold with coffee or tea.

Nutrition:
- Calories: 210
- Carbs: 4g
- Protein: 5g
- Fat: 18g

Ham and Spinach Frittata

Preparation time:

15 minutes

Cooking time:

2 hours

Servings:

4 people

Ingredients:

- 10 large eggs
- ½ diced green bell pepper, diced
- 1 cup of ham, diced
- 2 handfuls of fresh spinach
- Salt and pepper

Directions:

1. Put a parchment liner in your slow cooker and grease it with non-stick cooking spray.
2. Put the peppers, spinach, and ham into the slow cooker.
3. Whisk the eggs into your large bowl.
4. Add salt and pepper, and then pour the eggs into the slow cooker.

5. Cook the ingredients on high for 1 ½ to 2 hours.
6. Slice the frittata, divide onto plates, and serve.

Nutrition:
- Calories: 109
- Fat: 6.9g
- Carbs: 1.8g
- Protein: 5.6g

Cheese Grits

Preparation time:

5 minutes

Cooking time:

5-7 hours

Servings:

4 people

Ingredients:

- 1/2 cup stone-ground grits
- 5-6 cups of water
- 2 tsp salt
- 1/2 cup Cheddar cheese (shredded)
- 6 tbsp butter
- Black pepper (optionally)

Directions:

1. Preheat slow cooker on low, spray the dish with cooking spray, or cover with butter. In a wide bowl, mix grits and water, add salt. Cook on low temperatures for 5-7 hours; you can leave it overnight.
2. Remove the dish from the slow cooker, cover butter on top.

3. Stir with the whisk to an even consistency and fully melted butter.
4. To serve, sprinkle more cheese on top and black pepper to your taste.
5. Serve warm.

Nutrition:
- Calories: 173
- Fat: 7g
- Carbs: 4g
- Protein: 6g

Pineapple Cake with Pecans

Preparation time:

15 minutes

Cooking time:

3-4 hours

Servings:

4 people

Ingredients:

- 2 cups of sugar
- 2 cups plain flour
- 2 eggs
- 4 tbsp vegetable oil
- 1 can pineapple with juice (crushed)
- 1 tsp baking soda
- 1 tsp vanilla extract
- Salt

For icing:

- 1 cup of sugar
- 1/2 cup butter
- 6 tbsp evaporated milk
- 3 tbsp shredded coconut
- 1/2 cup chopped pecans (toasted)

Directions:

1. Preheat your slow cooker to 180-200°F. Take a medium bowl and combine all cake ingredients.
2. Mix the dough until evenly combined and then pour into slow cooker dish.
3. Bake for 3 hours on high; check if it is ready with a wooden toothpick.
4. When the cake is ready, make the icing: in a medium saucepan, combine sugar, evaporated milk, butter, and salt.
5. Bring to boil, and then simmer with a lower heat for 10 minutes.
6. Add the coconut to the icing.
7. Put the icing over the hot cake, then sprinkle with nuts.
8. To serve, let the cake cool, then cut it and serve with your favorite drinks.

Nutrition:

- Calories: 291
- Fat: 7g
- Carbs: 6g
- Protein: 5g

Potato Casserole for Breakfast

Preparation time:

5 minutes

Cooking time:

4 hours

Servings:

4 people

Ingredients:

- 4 big potatoes
- 5-6 sausages
- 1/2 cup cheddar cheese (shredded)
- 1/2 cup mozzarella cheese
- 5-6 green onions
- 10 chicken eggs
- 1/2 cup milk
- Salt
- Black pepper

Directions:

1. Preheat slow cooker on low; spray its dish with non-stick cooking spray. Rub the potatoes into small pieces and put them into the dish.

2. Cover the potatoes with rubbed sausages.
3. Add both mozzarella, cheddar cheeses, and green onions.
4. Continue the layers until all space in the dish is full.
5. Mix the wet ingredients (milk, eggs) in a medium bowl.
6. Pour it into the main dish, then put salt and pepper. Leave to cook on low for 5 hours or until the eggs are set.
7. Serve with guacamole or green onions.

Nutrition:
- Calories: 190
- Fat: 10g
- Carbs: 5g
- Protein: 10g

Cinnamon Rolls

Preparation time:

15 minutes

Cooking time:

2 hours

Servings:

10-12 pieces

Ingredients:

- 2 cups warm water
- 1 tbsp active yeast (dry)
- 2 tbsp wild honey
- 3 cups plain flour
- 1 tsp salt
- 4 tbsp butter
- 4 tbsp brown sugar
- 1 tsp cinnamon

Directions:

1. In a bowl, mix up water, yeast, and honey.
2. Stir with a mixer and after the dough is homogenous, let it rest for several minutes; mixture will rise.
3. Sift flour and add salt.

4. Mix on low to let the ingredients come together, then increase the mixing speed to medium.
5. Remove dough and allow to rise on a floured table.
6. Roll dough into medium rectangles. You can use a pizza cutter to make the sides even. Spread the butter over the dough. Sprinkle it with sugar and cinnamon.
7. Roll the dough rectangles into a long log, and then cut it into 10-12 pieces.
8. Cover your slow cooker inside with foil, place the rolls over it and cook on high for 2-3 hours.
9. To serve, use fresh berries or mint leaves.

Nutrition:
- Calories: 190
- Fat: 5g
- Carbs: 7g
- Protein: 8g

Quinoa Pie

Preparation time:

10 minutes

Cooking time:

4 hours

Servings:

4 people

Ingredients:

- 2 tbsp almond butter
- 2 tbsp maple syrup
- 1 cup vanilla almond milk
- 1 tsp salt
- 1/2 cup quinoa
- 2 chicken eggs
- Cinnamon
- 1/2 cup raisins
- 5 tbsp roasted almonds (chopped)
- 1/2 cup dried apples

Directions:

1. Spray the slow cooker dish with no-stick spray or cover it with foil or parchment paper.

2. In another bowl, mix the almond butter and maple syrup.
3. Melt in a microwave until creamy, about a minute.
4. Add almond milk, salt, and cinnamon, then whisk the mass until it is entirely even.
5. Add the eggs and remaining products, mix well. Preheat your slow cooker to 100-110°F.
6. Put the dough into the dish, then place it into the slow cooker.
7. Cook for 3-4 hours on high. To serve, remove the pie out of the dish with a knife.
8. Cool in the refrigerator.

Nutrition:

- Calories: 174
- Fat: 8g
- Carbs: 20g
- Protein: 6g

Quinoa Muffins with Peanut Butter

Preparation time:

10 minutes

Cooking time:

4 hours

Servings:

8 muffins

Ingredients:

- 1 cup strawberries
- 1/2 cup almond vanilla milk
- 1 tsp salt
- 5-6 tbsp raw quinoa
- 2 tbsp peanut butter (better natural)
- 3 tbsp honey
- 4 egg whites
- 2 tbsp peanuts (roasted)

Directions:

1. Preheat your slow cooker to 190°F. Line the cooking dish bottom with parchment paper; additionally, spray it with cooking spray. Dice the strawberries and place them over the dish.

2. Sprinkle with honey and place the dish into the slow cooker for 10-15 minutes for releasing juices. In another pot, mix up the almond milk and salt. Boil with quinoa until ready.
3. Combine egg whites and almond butter in a separate bowl. Put the quinoa and wait until milk is absorbed.
4. Fill the muffin forms with quinoa mixture; place the strawberries on the top. Bake in the slow cooker on low until quinoa is set for about 4 hours. To serve, cool the muffins and decorate them with whole strawberries.

Nutrition:
- Calories: 190
- Fat: 6 g
- Carbs: 8 g
- Protein: 6 g

Veggie Omelets

Preparation time:

5 minutes

Cooking time:

2 hours

Servings:

8 pieces

Ingredients:

- 6 chicken eggs
- 1/2 cup milk
- salt
- garlic powder
- white pepper
- red pepper
- small onion
- garlic clove
- parsley
- 5 small tomatoes

Directions:

1. Grease the slow cooker dish with butter or special cooking spray. In a separate bowl, mix up eggs and milk.

2. Add pepper and garlic.
3. Whisk the mixture well and salt. Add to the mixture broccoli florets, onions, pepper, and garlic. Stir in the eggs.
4. Place the mixture into the slow cooker dish.
5. Cook on high temperatures at 180-200°F for 2 hours.
6. Cover with cheese and let it melt.
7. To serve, cut the omelet into 8 pieces and garnish the plates with parsley and tomatoes.

Nutrition:
- Calories: 210
- Fat: 7 g
- Carbs: 5 g
- Protein: 8 g

Apple Pie with Oatmeal

Preparation time:

10 minutes

Cooking time:

4-6 hours

Servings:

4 people

Ingredients:

- 1 cup oats
- 2 large apples
- 2 cups almond milk
- 2 cups warm water
- 2 tsp cinnamon
- Pinch nutmeg
- Salt
- 2 tbsp coconut oil
- 1 tsp vanilla extract
- 2 tbsp flaxseeds
- 2 tbsp maple syrup
- Raisins

Directions:

1. Grease your slow cooker. Rub a couple of spoons of coconut or olive oil.
2. Peel the apples. Core and chop them into medium size pieces.
3. Starting with the apples, add all the ingredients into the slow cooker.
4. Stir and leave to bake for 6 hours on low. When ready, stir the oatmeal well.
5. Serve the oatmeal into small cups.
6. You can also garnish it with any berries or toppings you like.

Nutrition:

- Calories: 159
- Fat: 12g
- Carbs: 9g
- Protein: 28g

Vanilla French Toast

Preparation time:

15 minutes

Cooking time:

8 hours/overnight

Servings:

4 people

Ingredients:

- 1 loaf bread (better day-old)
- 2 cups cream
- 2 cups milk, whole
- 8 eggs
- almond extract
- 1 vanilla bean
- 5 tsp sugar
- Cinnamon
- Salt

Directions:

1. Coat the slow cooker dish with the cooking spray.
2. Slice bread into small pieces (1-2 inches).

3. Place them into the dish overlapping each other.
4. In another dish, combine the remaining ingredients until perfectly blended.
5. Pour the wet mixture over the bread to cover it completely.
6. Place the dish into a slow cooker and cook on low at 100-120°F for 7-8 hours.
7. To serve, slightly cool and cut the French toast.

Nutrition:
- Calories: 200
- Fat: 6g
- Carbs: 4g
- Protein: 8g

Greek Eggs Casserole

Preparation time:

15 minutes

Cooking time:

6 hours

Servings:

4 people

Ingredients:

- 10 chicken eggs
- 1/2 cup milk
- Salt
- 1 tsp black pepper
- 1 tbsp red onion
- 1/2 cup dried tomatoes
- 1 cup champignons
- 2cups spinach
- 1/2 cup feta

Directions:

1. Set your slow cooker to 120-150°F. In a separate wide bowl, combine and whisk the eggs.

2. Add salt and pepper. Mix in garlic and red onion. Whisk again.
3. Wash and dice the mushrooms.
4. Put them into the wet mixture.
5. At last, and add dried tomatoes.
6. Pour the mixture into the slow cooker.
7. Top the meal with the feta cheese and cook on low for 5-6 hours.
8. Serve with milk or vegetables.

Nutrition:
- Calories: 180
- Fat: 8 g
- Carbs: 4 g
- Protein: 8 g

Banana Bread

Preparation time:

15 minutes

Cooking time:

4 hours

Servings:

3 people

Ingredients:

- 2 chicken eggs
- 1/2 cup softened butter
- 1 cup of sugar
- 2 cups plain flour
- 1/2 teaspoon baking soda
- Salt
- 3 medium bananas

Directions:

1. First, cover with cooking spray and preheat your slow cooker.
2. Combine eggs with sugar and butter. Stir well.
3. Mix in baking soda and baking powder.
4. Peel and mash bananas, mix them with flour, and combine with eggs.

5. Pour the dough into the cooking dish and place it into the slow cooker.
6. Cook on low for 3-4 hours.
7. When ready, remove the bread with a knife and enjoy your breakfast!
8. To serve, use fresh bananas, apples, or berries to your taste.

Nutrition:

- Calories: 130
- Fat: 8g
- Carbs: 5g
- Protein: 7g

Treacle Sponge with Honey

Preparation time:

15 minutes

Cooking time:

3 hours

Servings:

4 people

Ingredients:

- 1 cup unsalted butter
- 3 tbsp. honey
- 1 tbsp. white breadcrumbs (fresh)
- 1 cup of sugar
- 1 lemon zest
- 3 large chicken eggs
- 2 cup flour
- 2 tbsp. milk
- Clotted cream (to serve)
- Little brandy splash (optional)

Directions:

1. Grease your slow cooker dish heavily and preheat it.

2. Mix the breadcrumbs with the honey in a medium bowl.
3. Melt butter and beat it with lemon zest and sugar until fluffy and light.
4. Sift in the flour slowly.
5. Add the milk and stir well. Spoon the mixture into the slow cooker dish.
6. Cook for 3 hours on low mode.
7. Serve with honey or clotted cream.

Nutrition:

- Calories: 200
- Fat: 10g
- Carbs: 20g
- Protein: 10g

Sticky Pecan Buns with Maple

Preparation time:

15 minutes

Cooking time:

5 hours

Servings:

12 rolls

Ingredients:

- 6 tbsp. milk (nonfat)
- 4 tbsp. maple syrup
- 1/2 tbsp. melted butter
- 1 tsp. vanilla extract
- Salt
- 2 tbsp. yeast
- 2 cup flour (whole wheat)
- Chopped pecans
- Ground cinnamon

Directions:

1. Coat the inside of your slow cooker using a non-stick cooking spray.
2. For the dough, combine milk, vanilla butter, and maple syrup. Mix well.

3. Microwave the mixture until warm and add the yeast. Let sit for 15 minutes.
4. Sift in the flour and mix until the dough is no stickier.
5. For the filling, mix the maple syrup and cinnamon.
6. Roll out the dough and brush it with the maple filling. Roll up, then slice into 10-12 parts. Place the small rolls into the slow cooker.
7. For the caramel sauce, combine milk, butter, and syrup.
8. Pour the sauce into the slow cooker.
9. Cook for 2 hours on high or 5 hours on low. Serve.

Nutrition:

- Calories: 230
- Fat: 5g
- Carbs: 29g
- Protein: 42g

Vegetarian Pot Pie

Preparation time:

15 minutes

Cooking time:

9 hours & 15 minutes

Servings:

4 people

Ingredients:

- 6 cups chopped vegetables (peas, potatoes, tomatoes, carrots, brussels sprouts)
- 1-2 cups diced mushrooms
- 2 onions
- 1/2 cup flour
- 4 cloves garlic
- 2 tbsp. garlic
- Thyme (fresh)
- Cornstarch
- 2 cups chicken broth

Directions:

1. Wash and chop vegetables or by frozen packed.
2. Toss with flour to cover vegetables well.

3. Mix with the broth slowly, when well combined with flour.
4. Preheat the slow cooker and place the vegetables into it.
5. Cook on low for 8-9 hours, or on high for 6-7 hours.
6. Mix up cornstarch with the water and pour into the vegetable mix.
7. Place it back in the slow cooker for 15 minutes. Serve hot with fresh vegetables.

Nutrition:
- Calories: 267
- Fat: 7g
- Carbs: 29g
- Protein: 7g

Blueberry Porridge

Preparation time:

5 minutes

Cooking time:

5-6 hours

Servings:

4 people

Ingredients:

- 1 cup jumbo oats
- 4 cups of milk
- 1/2 cup dried fruits
- Brown sugar or honey
- Cinnamon
- Blueberries

Directions:

1. Heat the slow cooker before the start.
2. Put the oats into the slow cooker dish, add some salt.
3. Pour over the milk, then place the dish into the slow cooker and cook on low for 7-8 hours (overnight).
4. Stir the porridge in the morning.

5. For serving, ladle into the serving bowls and decorate with your favorite yogurt or syrup. Add blueberries.

Nutrition:

- Calories: 210
- Fat: 4 g
- Carbs: 5 g
- Protein: 8 g

Cauliflower and Eggs Bowls

Preparation time:

15 minutes

Cooking time:

7 hours

Servings:

2 people

Ingredients:

- Cooking spray
- 4 eggs, whisked
- A pinch of salt and black pepper
- ¼ teaspoon thyme, dried
- ½ teaspoon turmeric powder
- 1 cup cauliflower florets
- ½ small yellow onion, chopped
- 3 oz. breakfast sausages, sliced
- ½ cup cheddar cheese, shredded

Directions:

1. Oiled your slow cooker with cooking spray and spread the cauliflower florets on the bottom of the pot.

2. Add the eggs mixed with salt, pepper, and the other ingredients and toss.
3. Put the lid on, cook on low for 7 hours, divide between plates, and serve for breakfast.

Nutrition:
- Calories: 261
- Fat: 6g
- Carbs: 22g
- Protein: 6g

Milk Oatmeal

Preparation time:

10 minutes

Cooking time:

2 hours

Servings:

4 people

Ingredients:

- 2 cups oatmeal
- 1 cup of water
- 1 cup milk
- 1 tablespoon liquid honey
- 1 teaspoon vanilla extract
- 1 tablespoon coconut oil
- ¼ teaspoon ground cinnamon

Directions:

1. Put all ingredients except liquid honey in the slow cooker and mix.
2. Cook the meal on high for hours.
3. Then stir the cooked oatmeal and transfer to the serving bowls.

4. Top the meal with a small amount of liquid honey.

Nutrition:
- Calories: 234
- Protein: 7.4 g
- Carbs: 35.3 g
- Fat: 7.3 g

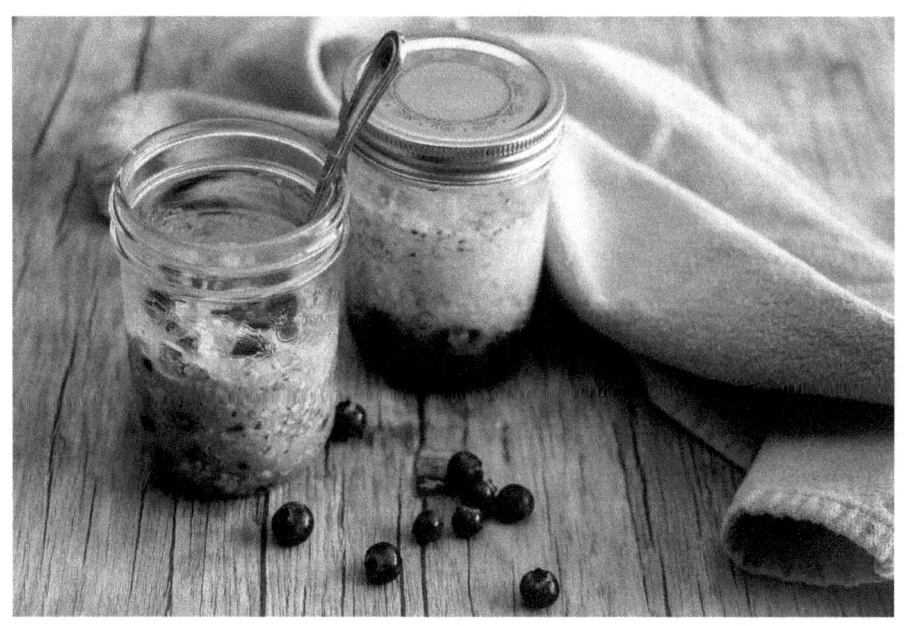

Asparagus Egg Casserole

Preparation time:

15 minutes

Cooking time:

2 hours & 30 minutes

Servings:

4 people

Ingredients:

- 7 eggs, beaten
- 4 oz asparagus, chopped, boiled
- 1 oz Parmesan, grated
- 1 teaspoon sesame oil
- 1 teaspoon dried dill

Directions:

1. Pour the sesame oil into the slow cooker.
2. Then mix dried dill with parmesan, asparagus, and eggs.
3. Pour the egg batter into your slow cooker and close the lid.
4. Cook the casserole on high for 2 hours and 30 minutes. Serve.

Nutrition:

- Calories: 149
- Protein: 12.6 g
- Carbs: 2.1 g
- Fat: 10.3 g

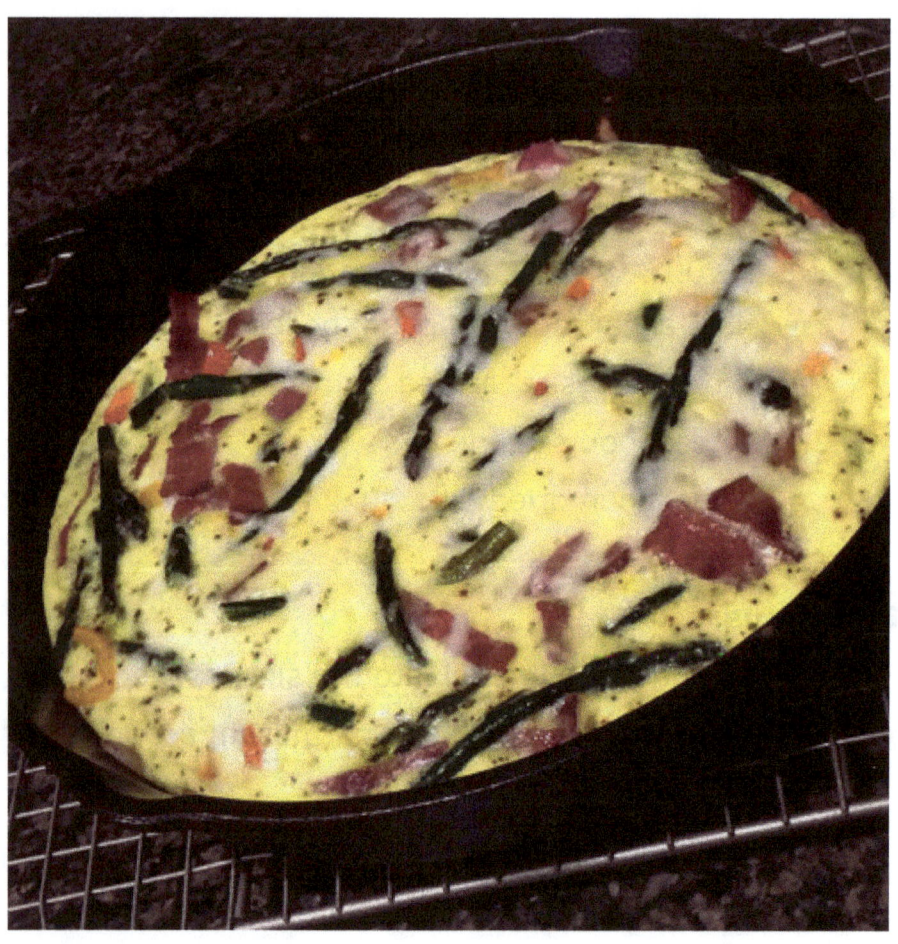

Vanilla Maple Oats

Preparation time:

15 minutes

Cooking time:

8 hours

Servings:

4 people

Ingredients:

- 1 cup steel-cut oats
- 2 tsp vanilla extract
- 2 cups vanilla almond milk
- 2 tbsp maple syrup
- 2 tsp cinnamon powder
- 2 cups of water
- 2 tsp flaxseed
- Cooking spray
- 2 tbsp blackberries

Directions:

1. Coat the base of your slow cooker with cooking spray.
2. Stir in oats, almond milk, vanilla extract, cinnamon, maple syrup, flaxseeds, and water.

3. Put the cooker's lid on and set the cooking time to 8 hours on low.
4. Stir well and serve with blackberries on top. Devour.

Nutrition:

- Calories: 200
- Fat: 3g
- Carbs: 9g
- Protein: 3g

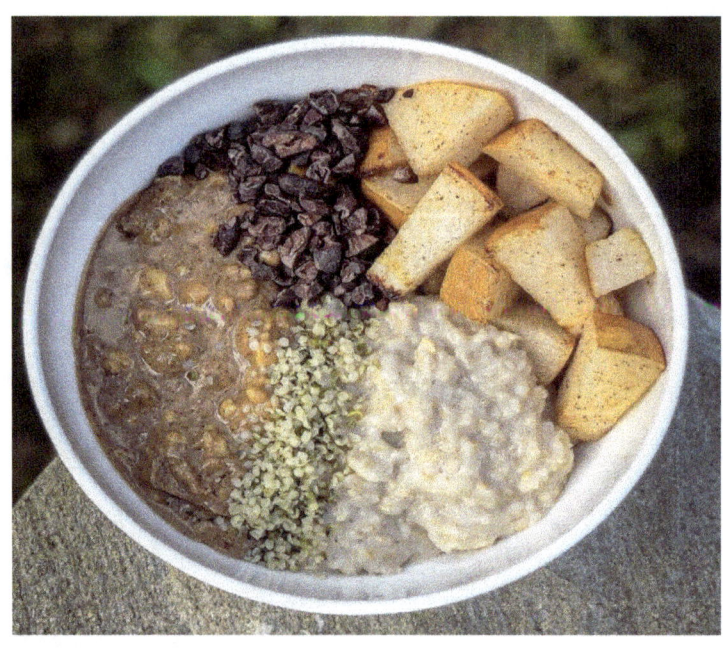

Raspberry Oatmeal

Preparation time:

15 minutes

Cooking time:

8 hours

Servings:

4 people

Ingredients:

- 2 cups of water
- 1 tablespoon coconut oil
- 1 cup steel-cut oats
- 1 tablespoon sugar
- 1 cup milk
- ½ teaspoon vanilla extract
- 1 cup raspberries
- 4 tablespoons walnuts, chopped

Directions:

1. In your slow cooker, mix oil with water, oats, sugar, milk, vanilla, and raspberries, cover, and cook on low for 8 hours.
2. Stir oatmeal, divide into bowls, sprinkle walnuts on top, and serve for breakfast.

Nutrition:

- Calories: 200
- Fat: 10 g
- Carbs: 20 g
- Protein: 4 g

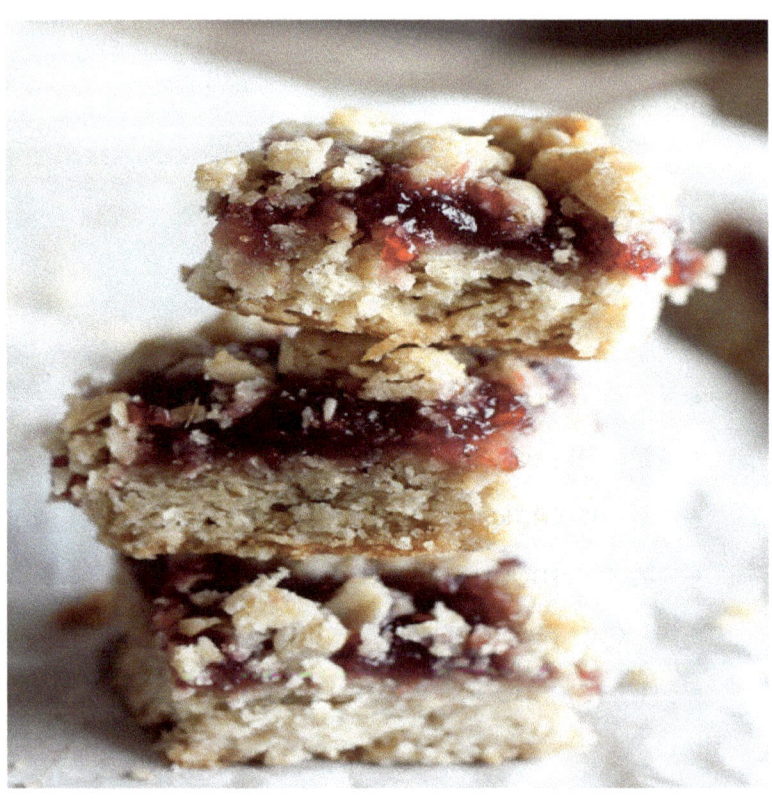

Pork and Eggplant Casserole

Preparation time:

15 minutes

Cooking time:

6 hours

Servings:

2 people

Ingredients:

- 1 red onion, chopped
- 1 eggplant, cubed
- ½ pound pork stew meat, ground
- 3 eggs, whisked
- ½ teaspoon chili powder
- ½ teaspoon garam masala
- 1 tablespoon sweet paprika
- 1 teaspoon olive oil

Directions:

1. Mix the eggs with the meat, onion, eggplant, and the other ingredients in the bowl except for the oil.

2. Grease your slow cooker with oil, add the pork and eggplant mix, spread into the pot, cook on low for 6 hours.
3. Divide the mixture between plates and serve for breakfast.

Nutrition:
- Calories: 261
- Fat: 7g
- Carbs: 16g
- Protein: 7g

Baby Spinach Rice Mix

Preparation time:

15 minutes

Cooking time:

6 hours

Servings:

4 people

Ingredients:

- ¼ cup mozzarella, shredded
- ½ cup baby spinach
- ½ cup wild rice
- 1 and ½ cups chicken stock
- ½ teaspoon turmeric powder
- ½ teaspoon oregano, dried
- A pinch of salt and black pepper
- 3 scallions, minced
- ¾ cup goat cheese, crumbled

Directions:

1. In your slow cooker, mix the rice with the stock, turmeric, and the other ingredients, toss, cook on low for 6 hours.

2. Divide the mix into bowls and serve for breakfast.

Nutrition:
- Calories: 165
- Fat: 1.2 g
- Carbs: 32.6 g
- Protein: 7.6 g

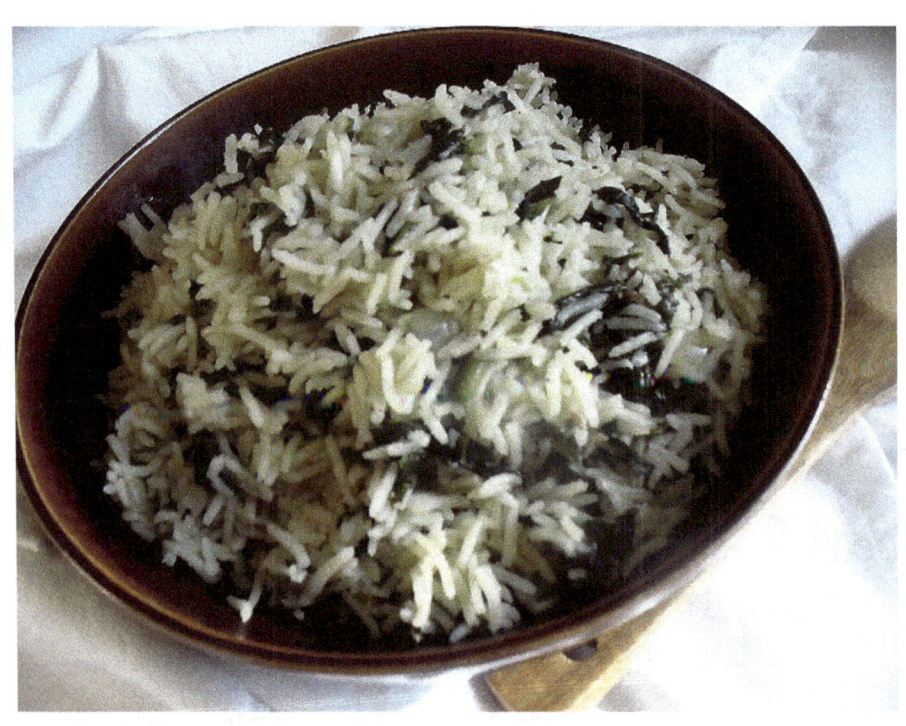

Baby Carrots in Syrup

Preparation time:

15 minutes

Cooking time:

7 hours

Servings:

4 people

Ingredients:

- 3 cups baby carrots
- 1 cup apple juice
- 2 tablespoons brown sugar
- 1 teaspoon vanilla extract

Directions:

1. Mix apple juice, brown sugar, and vanilla extract.
2. Pour the liquid into the slow cooker.
3. Add baby carrots and close the lid.
4. Cook the meal on low for 7 hours.

Nutrition:

- Calories: 81
- Protein: 0 g
- Carbs: 18.8 g
- Fat: 0.1 g

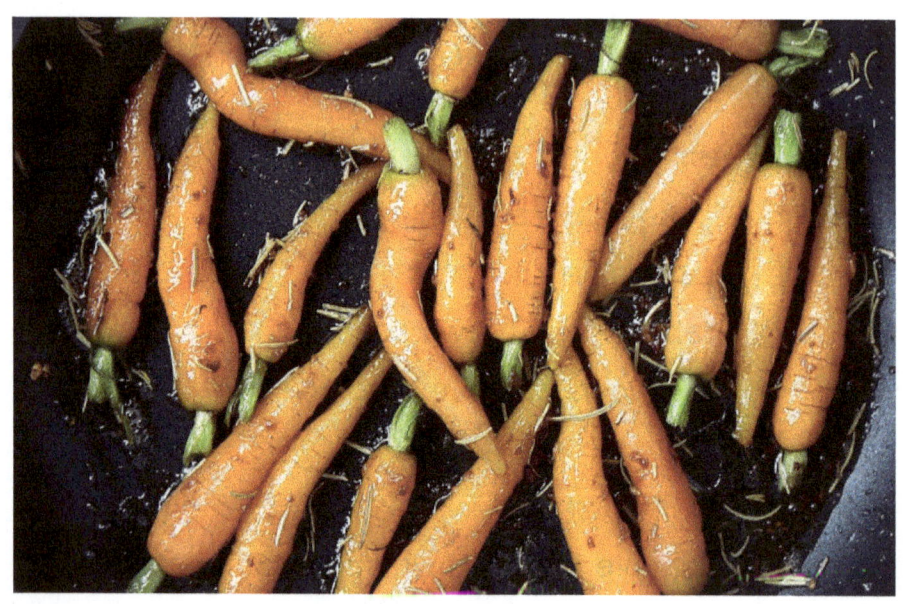

Green Muffins

Preparation time:

15 minutes

Cooking time:

2 hours & 30 minutes

Servings:

8 muffins

Ingredients:

- 1 cup spinach, washed
- 5 tbsp butter
- 1 cup flour
- 1 tsp salt
- ½ tsp baking soda
- 1 tbsp lemon juice
- 1 tbsp sugar
- 3 eggs

Directions:

1. Add the spinach leaves to a blender jug and blend until smooth.
2. Whisk the eggs in a bowl and add the spinach mixture.

3. Stir in baking soda, salt, sugar, flour, and lemon juice.
4. Mix well to form a smooth spinach batter. Divide the dough into a muffin tray lined with muffin cups.
5. Place this muffin tray in the slow cooker.
6. Put the cooker's lid on and set the cooking time to 2 hours 30 minutes on high.
7. Serve.

Nutrition:
- Calories: 172
- Fat: 6.1 g
- Carbs: 9.23 g
- Protein: 20 g

Scallions and Bacon Omelet

Preparation time:

15 minutes

Cooking time:

2 hours

Servings:

4 people

Ingredients:

- 5 eggs, beaten
- 2 oz bacon, chopped, cooked
- 1 oz scallions, chopped
- 1 teaspoon olive oil
- ½ teaspoon ground black pepper
- ¼ teaspoon cayenne pepper

Directions:

1. Brush the slow cooker bowl bottom with olive oil.
2. After this, mix eggs with bacon, scallions, ground black pepper, and cayenne pepper in the bowl.
3. Pour the liquid into your slow cooker and close the lid.

4. Cook the meal on high for 2 hours.
5. Serve.

Nutrition:
- Calories: 169
- Protein: 12.3g
- Carbs: 1.4g
- Fat: 12.6g

Cowboy Breakfast Casserole

Preparation time:

15 minutes

Cooking time:

3 hours

Servings:

4 people

Ingredients:

- 1-pound ground beef
- 5 eggs, beaten
- 1 cup grass-fed Monterey Jack cheese, shredded
- Salt and pepper to taste
- 1 avocado, peeled and diced
- A handful of cilantros, chopped
- A dash of hot sauce

Directions:

1. In a skillet over medium flame, sauté the beef for three minutes until slightly golden.
2. Pour into the slow cooker and pour in eggs.
3. Sprinkle with cheese on top and season with salt and pepper to taste.

4. Close the lid and cook on high for hours or on low for 6 hours.
5. Serve with avocado, cilantro, and hot sauce.

Nutrition:

- Calories: 439
- Carbs: 4.5 g
- Protein: 32.7 g
- Fat: 31.9 g

Maple Banana Oatmeal

Preparation time:

15 minutes

Cooking time:

6 hours

Servings:

2 people

Ingredients:

- 1/2 cup old fashioned oats
- 1 banana, mashed
- ½ teaspoon cinnamon powder
- 2 tablespoons maple syrup
- 2 cups almond milk
- Cooking spray

Directions:

1. Grease your slow cooker with the cooking spray, add the oats, banana, and the other ingredients, stir, cook on low for 6 hours.
2. Divide into bowls and serve for breakfast.

Nutrition:
- Calories: 815
- Fat: 60.3 g
- Carbs: 67 g
- Protein: 11.1 g

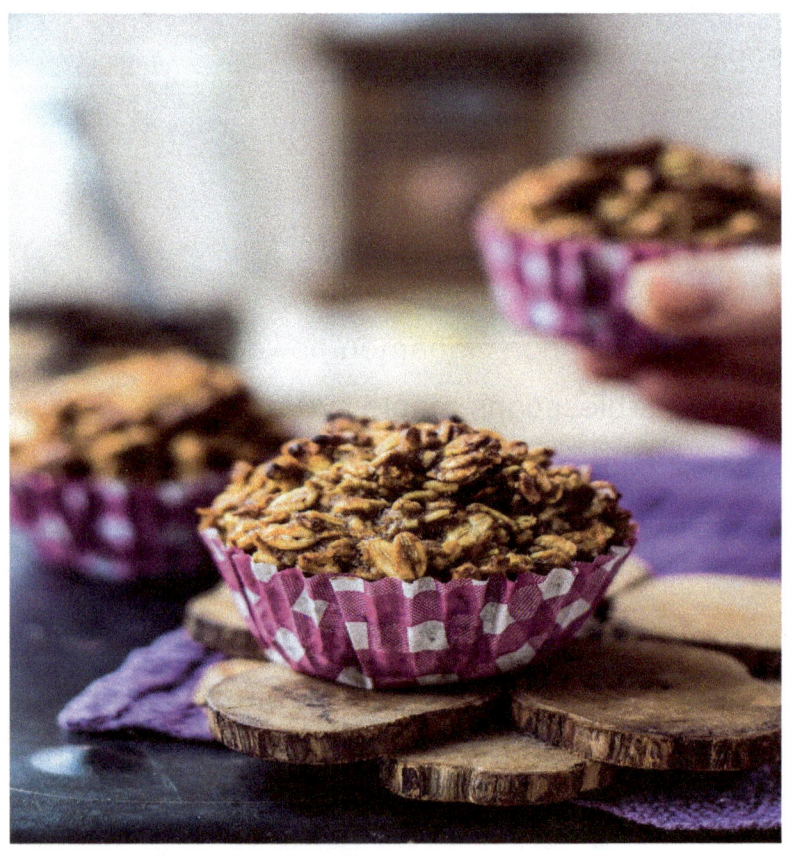

Potato Muffins

Preparation time:

15 minutes

Cooking time:

2 hours

Servings:

4 people

Ingredients:
- 4 teaspoons flax meal
- 1 bell pepper, diced
- 1 cup potato, cooked, mashed
- 2 eggs, beaten
- 1 teaspoon ground paprika
- 2 oz Mozzarella, shredded

Directions:
1. Mix flax meal with potato and eggs.
2. Then add ground paprika and bell pepper.
3. Stir the mixture with the help of the spoon until homogenous.
4. Transfer the potato mixture to the muffin molds.

5. Top the muffins with mozzarella and transfer them to the slow cooker.
6. Close the lid and cook the muffins on high for 2 hours.
7. Serve.

Nutrition:
- Calories: 107
- Protein: 8g
- Carbs: 7.2g
- Fat: 5.7g

Eggs and Sweet Potato Mix

Preparation time:

15 minutes

Cooking time:

6 hours

Servings:

2 people

Ingredients:

- ½ red onion, chopped
- ½ green bell pepper, chopped
- 2 sweet potatoes, peeled and grated
- ½ red bell pepper, chopped
- 1 garlic clove, minced
- ½ teaspoon olive oil
- 4 eggs, whisked
- 1 tablespoon chives, chopped
- A pinch of red pepper, crushed
- A pinch of salt and black pepper

Directions:

1. Mix the eggs with the onion, bell peppers, and the other ingredients in a bowl except for the oil.

2. Grease your slow cooker with the oil, add the eggs and potato mix, spread, cook on low within 6 hours.
3. Divide everything between plates and serve.

Nutrition:
- Calories: 261
- Fat: 6 g
- Carbs: 16 g
- Protein: 4 g

Veggie Hash Brown Mix

Preparation time:

15 minutes

Cooking time:

6 hours & 5 minutes

Servings:

2 people

Ingredients:

- 1 tablespoon olive oil
- ½ cup white mushrooms, chopped
- ½ yellow onion, chopped
- ¼ teaspoon garlic powder
- ¼ teaspoon onion powder
- ¼ cup sour cream
- 10 oz. hash browns
- ¼ cup cheddar cheese, shredded
- Salt and black pepper to the taste
- ½ tablespoon parsley, chopped

Directions:

1. Heat-up a pan with the oil over medium heat, add the onion and mushrooms, stir and cook for 5 minutes.

2. Transfer this to the slow cooker, add hash browns and the other ingredients, toss, cook on low within 6 hours.
3. Divide between plates and for breakfast.

Nutrition:
- Calories: 571
- Fat: 35.6g
- Carbs: 54.9g
- Protein: 9.7g

Coconut Cranberry Quinoa

Preparation time:

5 minutes

Cooking time:

2 hours

Servings:

4 people

Ingredients:

- 3 cups of coconut water
- 1 cup quinoa, uncooked and rinsed
- 3 teaspoons honey
- ¼ cup cranberries
- ½ cup coconut flakes

Directions:

1. Place all ingredients in the slow cooker.
2. Add a dash of vanilla or cinnamon if desired.
3. Give a good stir.
4. Cook on low within 2 hours. Serve.

Nutrition:

- Calories: 246
- Carbs: 42 g
- Protein: 8 g
- Fat: 5 g

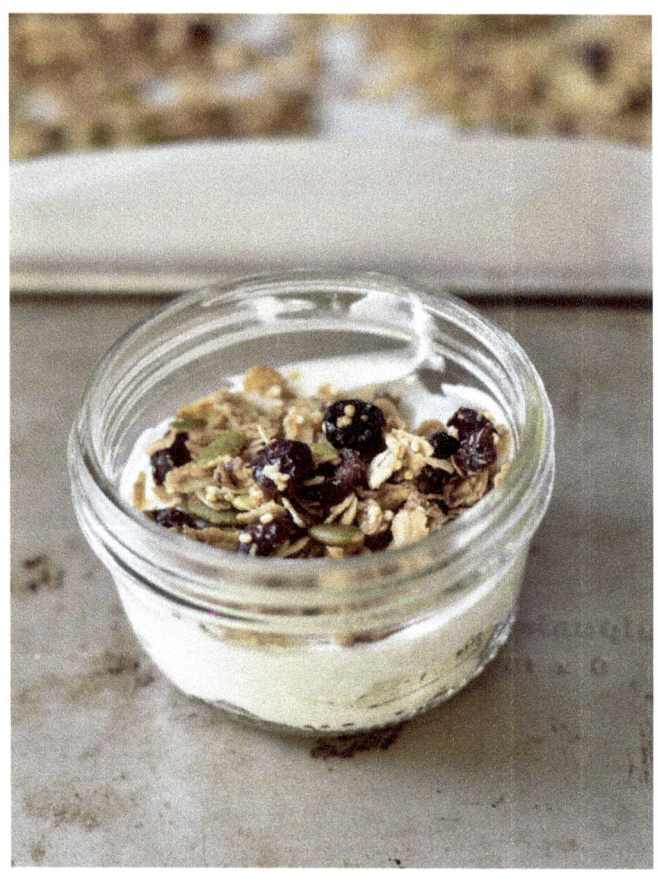

Scrambled Eggs in Ramekins

Preparation time:

5 minutes

Cooking time:

4 hours

Servings:

2 people

Ingredients:

- 2 eggs, beaten
- ¼ cup milk
- Salt and pepper
- ¼ cup cheddar cheese, grated
- ½ cup of salsa

Directions:

1. Mix the eggs and milk in a mixing bowl.
2. Season with salt and pepper to taste.
3. Place egg mixture in two ramekins.
4. Sprinkle with cheddar cheese on top.
5. Put the ramekins in the slow cooker, then pour water around it.
6. Cook on low within 4 hours.
7. Serve with salsa.

Nutrition:

- Calories: 243
- Carbs: 9.3 g
- Protein: 15.3 g
- Fat: 164 g

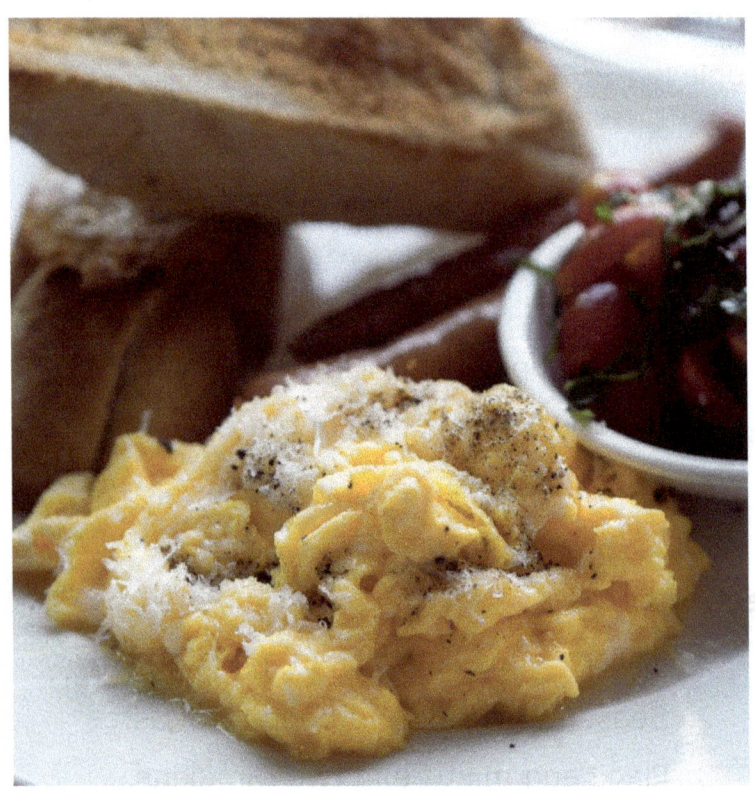

Enchilada Breakfast Casserole

Preparation time:

5 minutes

Cooking time:

10 hours

Servings:

4 people

Ingredients:

- 6 eggs, beaten
- 1-pound ground beef
- 2 cans enchilada sauce
- 1 can condensed cream of onion soup
- 3 cups sharp cheddar cheese, grated

Directions:

1. Beat the eggs, then season with salt plus pepper in a mixing bowl.
2. Set aside.
3. In a skillet, brown the beef for at least 5 minutes.
4. Pour the beef into the slow cooker and stir in the enchilada sauce and cream of onion soup. Stir in the eggs and place cheese on top.

5. Cook on low within 10 hours.
6. Serve.

Nutrition:
- Calories: 320
- Carbs: 9.4 g
- Protein: 24.6 g
- Fat: 20.1 g

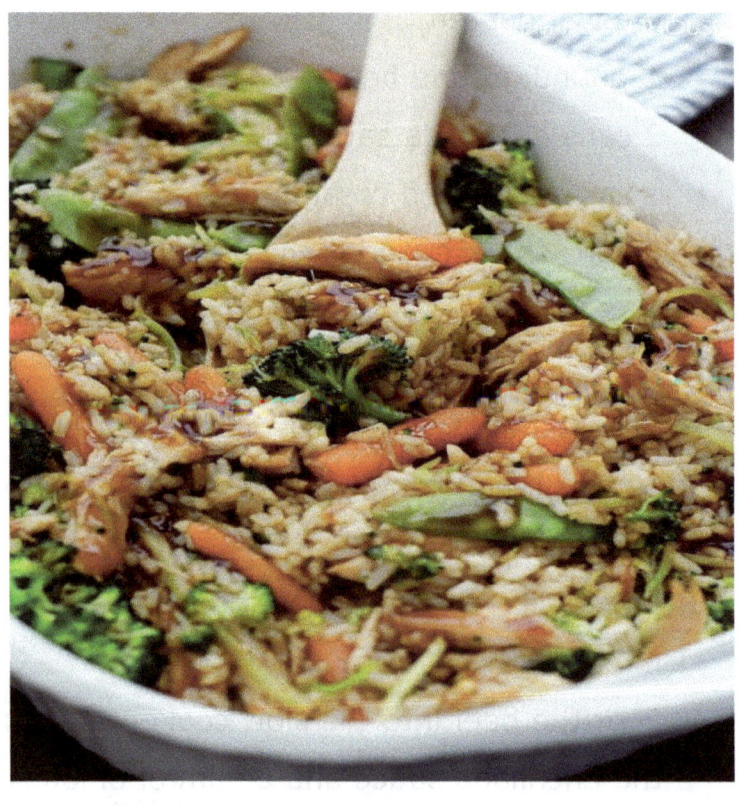

White Chocolate Oatmeal

Preparation time:

5 minutes

Cooking time:

4 hours

Servings:

4 people

Ingredients:

- 1 tablespoon white chocolate chips
- 1 cup of water
- ½ cup oatmeal
- 1 tablespoon brown sugar
- 1 teaspoon cinnamon

Directions:

1. Stir in all fixing in the slow cooker.
2. Cook on low within 4 hours.
3. Top with your favorite topping.

Nutrition:

- Calories: 31
- Carbs: 5.4 g

- Protein: 0.5 g
- Fat: 0.9 g

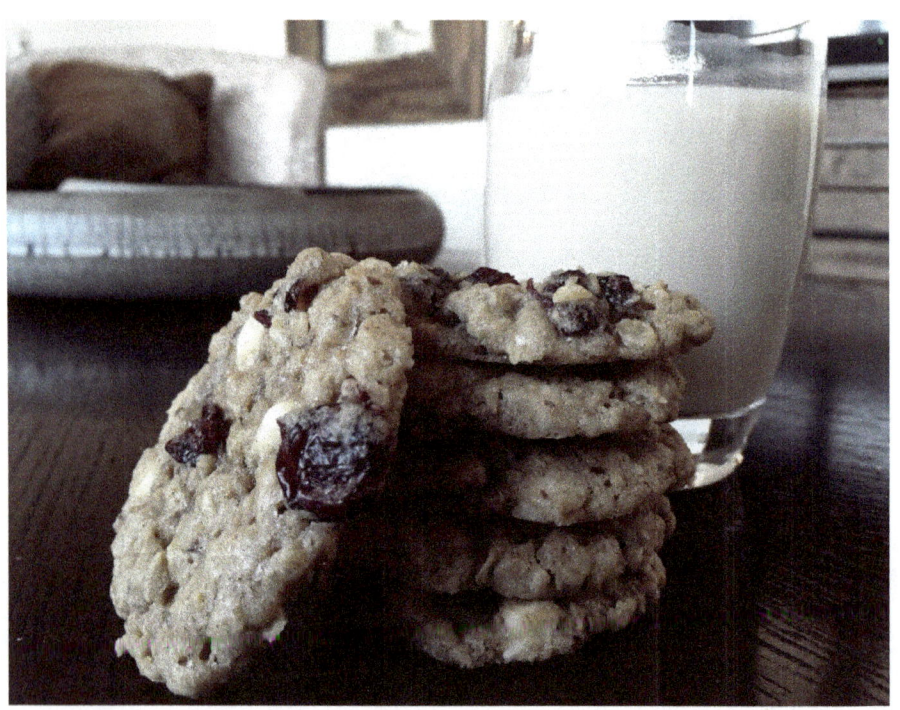

Bacon-Wrapped Hotdogs

Preparation time:

15 minutes

Cooking time:

8 hours

Servings:

4 people

Ingredients:

- 8 small hotdogs
- 8 bacon
- ½ cup brown sugar
- 4 tablespoons water
- Salt and pepper to taste

Directions:

1. Wrap the individual hotdogs with bacon strips. Secure with a toothpick, then place inside the slow cooker.
2. Mix the sugar, water, salt, and pepper in a small mixing bowl.
3. Pour over the hotdogs.
4. Cook on low within 8 hours.
5. Serve.

Nutrition:

- Calories: 120
- Carbs: 11.8 g
- Protein: 3.1 g
- Fat: 6.9 g

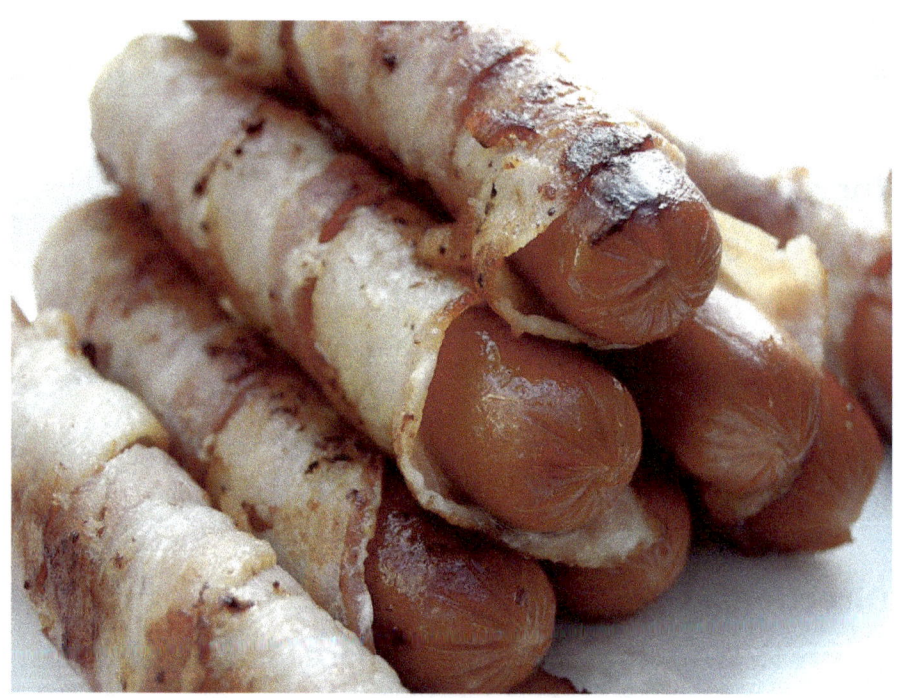

Apple Granola Crumble

Preparation time:

15 minutes

Cooking time:

3 hours

Servings:

4 people

Ingredients:

- 2 Granny Smith apples, cored and sliced
- 1 cup granola cereal
- 1/8 cup maple syrup
- ¼ cup apple juice
- 1 teaspoon cinnamon

Directions:

1. Place all ingredients in the slow cooker.
2. Give a good stir.
3. Cook on low within 3 hours.
4. Once cooked, serve with a tablespoon of butter.

Nutrition:

- Calories: 369
- Carbs: 56 g
- Protein: 5 g
- Fat:15 g

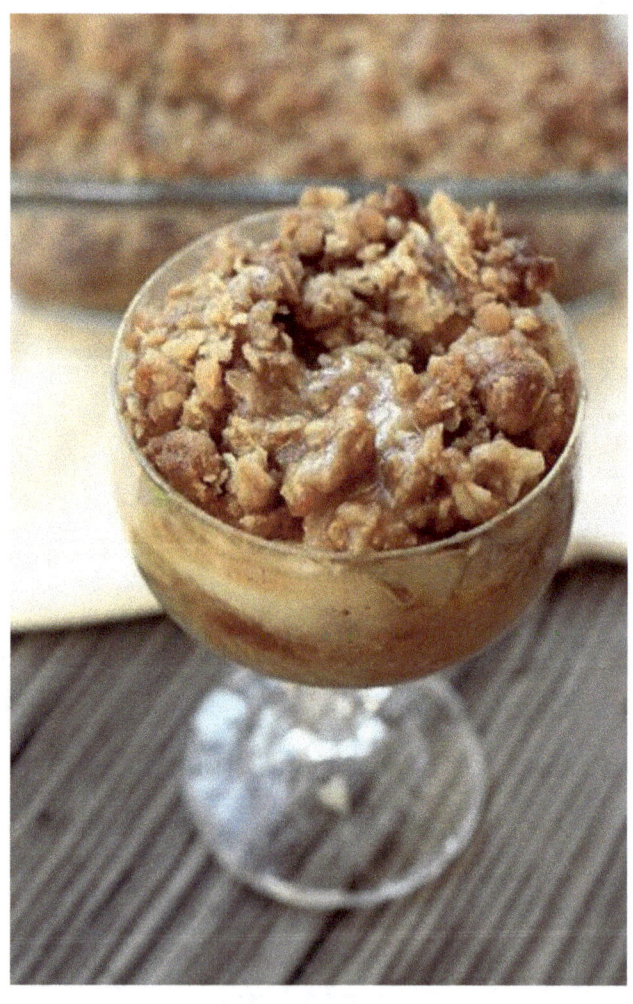

www.ingramcontent.com/pod-product-compliance
Lightning Source LLC
Chambersburg PA
CBHW070732030426
42336CB00013B/1951